INFECTIONS MED HANDBOOK

Bacterial Infections Treatment Secret Guide Using Augmentin

Dr. Amos Ben

Copyright@2024

Table of Contents

CHAPTER ONE 3

Introduction to Augmentin 4

CHAPTER TWO 11

Indications for using Augmentin 11

CHAPTER THREE 16

Augmentin Dosage and Administration 16

CHAPTER FOUR 22

Precautions and Contraindications of Augmentin 22

CHAPTER FIVE 28

Potential Side Effects of Augmentin 28

CHAPTER SIX 35

Drug Interactions with Augmentin 35

CHAPTER SEVEN..42

Monitoring and Follow-Up with Augmentin 42

CHAPTER EIGHT 48

Storage and Handling of Augmentin 48

CHAPTER NINE 53

Conclusion and Summary. 53

CHAPTER ONE

Introduction to Augmentin

Augmentin is a commonly given antibiotic that falls under the category of combination medicines. Its unique mixture contains two active ingredients: amoxicillin and clavulanic acid. This potent mixture increases its effectiveness against a wide range of bacterial illnesses.

Composition

Amoxicillin: Amoxicillin, a penicillin-type antibiotic, inhibits the production of bacterial cell walls, resulting in the bacteria's death.

Clavulanic acid is a beta-lactamase inhibitor.

Beta-lactamases are enzymes generated by some bacteria that may make medicines such as amoxicillin ineffective. Clavulanic acid helps to avoid this resistance mechanism, broadening the range of bacterial coverage.

Mechanism of Action.

Amoxicillin inhibits the production of the bacterial cell wall, weakening it and causing the bacterium to burst.

Clavulanic acid protects amoxicillin against breakdown by beta-lactamases, enzymes that certain bacteria manufacture to resist antibiotics. Augmentin's dual action mechanism makes it effective against a larger spectrum of microorganisms.

Application Indications

Augmentin is given to treat a variety of bacterial illnesses that affect different bodily systems.

Common indications include respiratory system infections (sinusitis, bronchitis, pneumonia), ear infections, urinary tract infections, skin and soft tissue infections, dental infections, bacterial sinusitis, and bone infections.

Formulations

Augmentin is available in a variety of formats, including pills, chewable tablets, and oral solution.

The formulation used is determined by the patient's age, weight, and the severity of the illness.

Dosages and Administration

The dose of Augmentin is determined on the particular illness, patient age, and weight.

It is often given orally and should be taken with meals to improve absorption and reduce gastrointestinal adverse effects.

Cautions and Contraindications

Patients who are allergic to penicillin or cephalosporin antibiotics should take care.

Individuals having a history of liver disease or jaundice may need an alternate therapy.

Potential Side Effects

Common adverse effects include nausea, vomiting, diarrhea, rash, stomach discomfort, and headache.

Serious adverse effects are uncommon, although they might include severe diarrhea, allergic reactions, and liver issues.

Drug interactions

Augmentin may interfere with other drugs, therefore patients should advise their doctor about any current prescriptions, supplements, or herbal preparations.

Monitoring and Follow-up

Patients should be followed for indications of improvement, and it is critical to finish the whole course of antibiotics as directed.

Any worrying side effects should be immediately reported to your healthcare physician.

Storage and Handling

Proper storage, particularly protection from moisture and heat, is critical for preserving the medication's efficacy.

The oral suspension has strict storage requirements, and any leftover medicine should be disposed of properly.

In summary, Augmentin is a flexible and strong antibiotic that is often used to treat bacterial infections.

Understanding its composition, mechanism of action, indications, dose, precautions, and possible adverse effects is critical for both healthcare practitioners and patients in order to deliver effective and safe therapy.

CHAPTER TWO

Indications for using Augmentin

Augmentin is a combination antibiotic that contains amoxicillin and clavulanic acid and is used to treat a wide range of bacterial infections affecting various organ systems in the body. Understanding its indications of use is critical for healthcare practitioners to prescribe the medicine correctly and for patients to understand when it may be required.

Respiratory Tract Infections

Augmentin is often used to treat respiratory tract infections, including:

Sinusitis: Inflammation of the sinuses, usually caused by bacterial infections.

Bronchitis is an inflammation of the bronchial passages that is usually caused by bacteria.

Pneumonia is an infection of the lungs caused by a variety of bacteria.

Middle ear infection, often known as otitis media, is a frequent bacterial illness in both adults and children. Augmentin is often recommended to treat acute otitis media and chronic ear infections.

Augmentin may cure simple urinary tract infections produced by susceptible bacteria.

Augmentin may be used to treat bacterial infections of the skin, including cellulitis and impetigo.

Augmentin is an effective treatment for dental infections, including abscesses caused by tooth decay or trauma.

For chronic or severe episodes of bacterial sinusitis, Augmentin therapy may be necessary to relieve symptoms and eliminate infection.

Augmentin may help treat osteomyelitis, a dangerous bone infection caused by bacteria.

Augmentin may be used for other bacterial illnesses, as determined by the healthcare professional, in addition to those mentioned above.

It's worth noting that Augmentin is ineffective against viral illnesses like the common cold or flu. Healthcare practitioners should undertake a comprehensive examination to identify whether the illness is bacterial in origin and whether Augmentin is the best antibiotic option depending on the susceptibility of the bacteria involved.

To summarize, Augmentin's indications for usage include a broad spectrum of bacterial diseases involving many organ systems. Understanding these indications enables healthcare practitioners to make more educated treatment choices, while also empowering patients to understand when Augmentin may be required for bacterial infections.

CHAPTER THREE

Augmentin Dosage and Administration

Proper dosage and administration of Augmentin are important for achieving optimal therapeutic outcomes while minimizing the risk of adverse effects and antibiotic resistance. Stated below are detailed steps for the dosage and administration of Augmentin.

Consultation with Healthcare Provider:

Before starting Augmentin therapy, patients should consult their healthcare provider. The provider will assess the nature and severity of the infection and determine if Augmentin is the appropriate treatment.

Determination of Dosage:

The dosage of Augmentin varies based on factors such as the type and severity of the infection, patient age, weight, and renal function.

The healthcare provider will calculate the appropriate dosage regimen for the patient.

Selection of Formulation:

Augmentin is available in various formulations, including tablets, chewable tablets, and oral suspension.

The choice of formulation depends on the patient's age, ability to swallow tablets, and the severity of the infection.

Administration with Food:

Augmentin drug should be taken with food to enhance absorption and reduce the risk of gastrointestinal upset. Patients should follow the instructions provided by their healthcare provider or pharmacist regarding the timing of doses with meals.

Tablet Administration:

If the prescribed formulation is tablets, patients should swallow the tablets whole with a full glass of water.

Patients should not crush or chew the tablets unless specifically instructed by their healthcare provider.

Chewable Tablet Administration:

Chewable tablets should be chewed thoroughly before swallowing.

Patients should follow the instructions provided by their healthcare provider or pharmacist regarding dosage and administration.

Preparation of Oral Suspension:

If the prescribed formulation is oral suspension, patients or caregivers should shake the bottle well before each use to ensure uniform distribution of the medication.

The oral suspension should be measured using a calibrated dosing device provided with the medication.

Storage of Oral Suspension:

The oral suspension may require refrigeration, depending on the specific formulation.

Patients should follow the storage instructions provided by their pharmacist or healthcare provider.

Completion of Full Course:

Patients should complete the full course of Augmentin as prescribed by their healthcare provider, even if symptoms improve before the medication is finished.

Premature discontinuation of antibiotics can lead to treatment failure and the development of antibiotic-resistant bacteria.

Monitoring and Follow-Up:

Patients should be monitored for signs of improvement in their symptoms and any potential adverse effects of Augmentin therapy.

Healthcare providers may schedule follow-up appointments to assess treatment response and adjust the treatment regimen if necessary.

proper dosage and administration of Augmentin involve careful consideration of the patient's clinical condition, appropriate selection of formulation, administration with food, and completion of the full course of treatment. Patients should adhere to the instructions provided by their healthcare provider or pharmacist to ensure the safe and effective use of Augmentin.

CHAPTER FOUR

Precautions and Contraindications of Augmentin

Augmentin like any other medication, carries certain precautions and contraindications that patients and healthcare providers should be aware of to ensure safe and effective use. Understanding these precautions and contraindications helps minimize the risk of adverse effects and complications. Stated below is a comprehensive explanation.

Allergy to Penicillin or Cephalosporins:

Patients with a known allergy to penicillin or cephalosporin antibiotics may be at increased risk of allergic reactions to Augmentin.

It's essential for patients to inform their healthcare provider of any known allergies before starting Augmentin therapy.

History of Severe Allergic Reactions:

Patients with a history of severe allergic reactions (anaphylaxis) to any medication should exercise caution when taking Augmentin.

Healthcare providers may opt for alternative antibiotics in patients with a history of severe allergic reactions.

Liver Problems or Jaundice:

Augmentin contains clavulanic acid, which can affect liver function in some individuals.

Patients with a history of liver problems or jaundice should use Augmentin cautiously under close medical supervision.

Renal Impairment:

Patients with renal impairment may require dosage adjustments or closer monitoring while taking Augmentin.

Healthcare providers should assess renal function before initiating Augmentin therapy and adjust the dosage accordingly.

Gastrointestinal Conditions:

Patients with a history of gastrointestinal disorders, such as colitis or inflammatory bowel disease, may experience exacerbation of symptoms while taking Augmentin.

Healthcare providers should evaluate the risks and benefits of Augmentin therapy in patients with pre-existing gastrointestinal conditions.

Pregnancy and Breastfeeding:

Augmentin is generally considered safe to use during pregnancy when the potential benefits outweigh the risks.

However, pregnant women should consult their healthcare provider before taking Augmentin.

Augmentin can pass into breast milk, so breastfeeding mothers should also consult their healthcare provider before taking the medication.

Interactions with Other Medications:

Augmentin may interact with certain medications, including oral contraceptives, anticoagulants, and probenecid.

Patients should inform their healthcare provider of all medications, supplements, and herbal products they are taking before starting Augmentin therapy.

Development of Antibiotic Resistance:

Overuse or misuse of antibiotics, including Augmentin, can contribute to the development of antibiotic resistance.

Healthcare providers should prescribe Augmentin only when necessary and educate patients about the importance of completing the full course of treatment.

Augmentin has several precautions and contraindications that patients and healthcare providers should be mindful of to ensure safe and effective use. Patients should inform their healthcare provider of any medical conditions, allergies, or medications they are taking before starting Augmentin therapy. Healthcare providers should evaluate the individual patient's risk factors and make informed decisions regarding the use of Augmentin based on the patient's clinical condition and medical history.

CHAPTER FIVE

Potential Side Effects of Augmentin

Augmentin like other medications, may cause side effects in some patients. Understanding these potential side effects is essential for both patients and healthcare providers to monitor for adverse reactions and take appropriate action if necessary. Stated below are comprehensive explanations of the potential side effects of Augmentin.

Nausea and Vomiting:

Nausea and vomiting are common side effects of Augmentin therapy.

Patients can take Augmentin with food to help minimize gastrointestinal discomfort.

Diarrhea:

Diarrhea is another common side effect of Augmentin, particularly in children.

Patients should stay hydrated and inform their healthcare provider if diarrhea is severe or persistent.

Rash:

Some patients may develop a rash or skin irritation while taking Augmentin.

It's essential to differentiate between a mild rash and a severe allergic reaction. Patients should seek medical attention if a rash is accompanied by other symptoms such as swelling, difficulty breathing, or fever.

Abdominal Pain:

Abdominal pain or discomfort may occur as a side effect of Augmentin.

Patients should inform their healthcare provider if abdominal pain is severe or persistent.

Headache:

Headaches are reported by some patients taking Augmentin.

Patients can try over-the-counter pain relievers with their healthcare provider's approval if headaches become bothersome.

Allergic Reactions:

Allergic reactions to Augmentin can range from mild to severe and may include hives, itching, swelling, and difficulty breathing.

Patients should seek immediate medical attention if they experience signs of a severe allergic reaction.

Severe Diarrhea or Colitis:

Augmentin use may lead to severe diarrhea or colitis (inflammation of the colon) in some patients.

Patients should stop taking Augmentin and contact their healthcare provider if they experience severe or persistent diarrhea, abdominal cramping, or bloody stools.

Liver Problems:

Augmentin contains clavulanic acid, which can cause liver problems in some individuals.

Patients should seek medical attention if they experience symptoms of liver problems, such as jaundice (yellowing of the skin or eyes), dark urine, or persistent fatigue.

Clostridium difficile Infection:

Augmentin use can disrupt the normal balance of bacteria in the intestines and increase the risk of Clostridium difficile infection, a serious and potentially life-threatening condition.

Patients should be vigilant for symptoms of C. difficile infection, including severe diarrhea, abdominal pain, and fever, and seek prompt medical attention if these symptoms occur.

Other Adverse Reactions:

Other less common side effects of Augmentin may include dizziness, insomnia, and changes in taste or smell.

Patients should report any unusual or bothersome symptoms to their healthcare provider.

Augmentin may cause a range of potential side effects, from mild gastrointestinal symptoms to severe allergic reactions and liver problems. Patients should be aware of these potential side effects and communicate any concerns or adverse reactions to their healthcare provider promptly.

Healthcare providers should monitor patients closely for side effects during Augmentin therapy and take appropriate measures to manage symptoms and ensure patient safety.

CHAPTER SIX

Drug Interactions with Augmentin

Drug interactions with Augmentin are very important for both healthcare providers and patients to ensure the safe and effective use of the medication. Drug interactions can impact the effectiveness of Augmentin or increase the risk of adverse effects. Stated below are drug interactions associated with Augmentin.

Probenecid:

Probenecid, a medication used to treat gout, can inhibit the renal excretion of Augmentin, leading to increased blood levels of the antibiotic.

Healthcare providers may adjust the dosage of Augmentin when co-administered with probenecid to prevent potential toxicity.

Oral Contraceptives:

Augmentin may reduce the effectiveness of oral contraceptives (birth control pills) by interfering with their absorption and metabolism.

Patients using hormonal contraceptives should consider using alternative or additional contraceptive methods while taking Augmentin to prevent unintended pregnancy.

Anticoagulants (Blood Thinners):

Augmentin may potentiate the effects of anticoagulant medications such as warfarin, increasing the risk of bleeding.

Healthcare providers may monitor the patient's international normalized ratio (INR) more closely when Augmentin is co-administered with anticoagulants and adjust the anticoagulant dosage as needed.

Methotrexate:

Concurrent use of Augmentin and methotrexate, a medication used to treat certain cancers and autoimmune diseases, may increase the risk of methotrexate toxicity.

Healthcare providers may monitor methotrexate levels and renal function more closely when these medications are used together.

Allopurinol:

Augmentin may increase the risk of allergic skin reactions when used concomitantly with allopurinol, a medication used to treat gout.

Patients should be monitored for signs of allergic reactions, and the medications may need to be adjusted or discontinued if necessary.

Proton Pump Inhibitors (PPIs) and H2 Blockers:

Proton pump inhibitors (PPIs) and H2 blockers, commonly used to treat gastroesophageal reflux disease (GERD) and peptic ulcers, may reduce the absorption of Augmentin.

Patients should avoid taking Augmentin with these medications if possible. If co-administration is necessary, the healthcare provider may adjust the timing of doses or recommend alternative therapies.

Other Antibiotics:

Concurrent use of Augmentin with other antibiotics, especially those with similar mechanisms of action or adverse effect profiles, may increase the risk of adverse reactions or antibiotic resistance.

Healthcare providers should carefully consider the risks and benefits of combining antibiotics and monitor patients closely for adverse effects.

Other Medications:

Augmentin may interact with various other medications, supplements, and herbal products. Patients should inform their healthcare provider of all medications they are taking, including over-the-counter drugs and herbal supplements, to avoid potential interactions.

Augmentin can interact with several medications, potentially affecting their efficacy or safety.

Healthcare providers should carefully evaluate the patient's medication regimen and consider potential drug interactions before prescribing Augmentin. Patients should also communicate any changes in their medication regimen to their healthcare provider to prevent adverse effects or treatment failures. Close monitoring and appropriate adjustments are essential to ensure the safe and effective use of Augmentin in clinical practice.

CHAPTER SEVEN

Monitoring and Follow-Up with Augmentin

Monitoring and follow-up are key components of Augmentin treatment to guarantee pharmaceutical efficacy, detect unwanted effects, and improve patient safety. The monitoring and follow-up stages for Augmentin therapy are outlined.

Initial Assessment:

The healthcare professional does an initial evaluation to determine the patient's medical history, including allergies, underlying health issues, and prior antibiotic usage.

In addition, the clinician evaluates the type and severity of the illness to decide the best course of Augmentin therapy.

Prescription and instructions:

When Augmentin is prescribed, the healthcare professional gives the patient precise information about the dose, administration, and length of the therapy.

Patients should carefully adhere to these directions and ask any concerns they may have regarding the drug.

Monitor your symptoms while using Augmentin. Improvement in symptoms, such as fever resolution, pain relief, or respiratory improvement, suggests a good response to therapy.

Patients should notify their healthcare practitioner as soon as any of their symptoms intensify or become new.

Monitor for side effects of Augmentin, including nausea, vomiting, diarrhea, rash, or stomach discomfort.

Patients should instantly notify their healthcare practitioner if they have any side effects.

Healthcare practitioners may plan follow-up consultations to assess patients' reaction to Augmentin medication.

During follow-up sessions, the physician reviews the patient's symptoms, assesses therapy response, and looks for any side effects or consequences.

Laboratory monitoring may be essential to evaluate a patient's response to Augmentin medication or identify possible side effects.

Blood tests, renal function tests, liver function tests, and complete blood counts may be ordered depending on the patient's clinical status and risk factors.

Patients with reduced renal function may need additional monitoring during Augmentin treatment to avoid drug buildup and toxicity.

Augmentin dose may be adjusted by healthcare practitioners depending on the patient's renal function, and renal function parameters should be monitored during therapy.

To ensure effective treatment, patients should finish the entire course of Augmentin given by their healthcare professional, even if symptoms improve before completion.

Premature antibiotic cessation may result in treatment failure and the growth of antibiotic-resistant microorganisms.

Patients undergoing Augmentin treatment should get continual instruction on drug adherence, possible adverse effects, and recovery strategies.

Patients should be encouraged to ask inquiries and express any concerns or challenges to their healthcare professional.

Monitoring and follow-up are critical components of Augmentin therapy to achieve the best treatment results and patient safety. Patients should take an active role in their treatment by monitoring their symptoms, reporting side effects, and attending follow-up visits as planned. Healthcare professionals play a vital role in monitoring therapy response, identifying side effects, and making any changes to the treatment plan. Close coordination between patients and healthcare professionals is essential for effective Augmentin treatment.

CHAPTER EIGHT

Storage and Handling of Augmentin

Augmentin should be stored and handled properly to ensure its stability, efficacy, and safety. The Augmentin storage and handling instructions are stated.

Storage temperature

Augmentin should be kept at room temperature, commonly between 68°F and 77°F (20°C to 25°C).

Avoid severe heat or cold, since these extremes might deteriorate the drug.

To prevent moisture and light exposure, keep Augmentin tablets and oral solution in a firmly sealed container.

Keep the medicine out of direct sunlight and moisture sources, such as restrooms and kitchen sinks.

refrigerated of Augmentin Oral Suspension: Some formulations may need refrigerated for stability.

Check the drug label or package insert for precise storage recommendations. Refrigerated suspension should be destroyed after a certain time, often 7 to 10 days.

Avoid freezing Augmentin oral solution or pills as it might affect their composition and efficacy.

Keep out of reach of children.

Augmentin should be stored in a safe area away from children and pets.

Accidental Augmentin consumption by children or pets may result in significant side effects that need rapid medical intervention.

Store Augmentin apart from other drugs, household chemicals, and food to avoid cross-contamination.

It is critical to retain Augmentin in its original package to prevent misunderstanding with other drugs.

To safely dispose of unused or expired Augmentin, follow local legislation and standards.

Do not flush or pour drugs down the drain unless directed to do so by specific disposal instructions or local rules.

Before using Augmentin, check the expiry date on the container.

Expired medicine may be ineffective or dangerous to use and should be disposed carefully.

Travel considerations:

When traveling with Augmentin, keep the drug in a cool, dry area out of direct sunlight and excessive temperatures.

If the oral suspension requires refrigeration, consider utilizing a travel cooler or an insulated bag.

Consult a healthcare provider or pharmacist:

If you have any questions or concerns about how to store and use Augmentin, talk to your doctor or pharmacist.

Healthcare experts and pharmacists may provide particular recommendations depending on the Augmentin formulation and unique storage circumstances.

Augmentin should be stored and handled properly to ensure its stability and efficacy. Patients should keep Augmentin at room temperature, away from moisture and light, and according to any particular storage instructions supplied by their healthcare professional or pharmacist. By following these suggestions, patients may ensure that Augmentin is used safely and effectively to treat bacterial infections.

CHAPTER NINE

Conclusion and Summary.

Augmentin is a combination antibiotic including amoxicillin and clavulanic acid, is a useful drug for treating a variety of bacterial infections. Throughout this thorough guide, we have covered Augmentin's indications, dosage and administration, precautions, possible adverse effects, medication interactions, monitoring and follow-up, and storage and handling requirements.

Augmentin is used to treat respiratory tract infections, ear infections, bladder infections, skin and soft tissue infections, dental infections, bacterial sinusitis, and bone infections.

It is available in a variety of forms, including tablets, chewable tablets, and oral suspensions, with doses based on the patient's age, weight, and infection severity.

Patients should be advised that possible side effects include nausea, vomiting, diarrhea, rash, stomach discomfort, headache, and allergic reactions. Close monitoring for adverse effects, as well as early reporting to healthcare practitioners, are critical to ensuring patient safety.

Drug interactions with Augmentin, including probenecid, oral contraceptives, anticoagulants, and others, may impair the medication's effectiveness and safety.

To prevent possible interactions, patients should notify their healthcare providers about any drugs, vitamins, and herbal preparations that they are using.

Monitoring and follow-up are essential components of Augmentin treatment, and include frequent symptom assessments, adverse effect monitoring, and laboratory testing as needed. To optimize treatment efficacy and reduce the possibility of antibiotic resistance, patients should take Augmentin for the whole period as advised.

Proper storage and handling of Augmentin, including protection from moisture and light, prevention of freezing, and adherence to storage temperature guidelines, are critical for medicine stability and efficacy.

In conclusion, Augmentin is an excellent antibiotic drug for treating a variety of bacterial illnesses. Patients and healthcare professionals should collaborate to ensure Augmentin is used safely and effectively, which includes adhering to recommended doses, monitoring for side effects, and following correct storage and handling procedures.

Following these recommendations allows patients to get the best therapeutic results while limiting the hazards associated with Augmentin medication.